Module Three

ISBN-13: 978-1984988935

A Working to Recovery Training & Education Pack

Devised and Edited by

Ron Coleman

Individuals who are interested in developing their own or their workforce skills in working with distressing voices have designed this training manual for use both by trainers, and. The manual is divided into a number of sections and covers the following:

1.   Background and potted history of the hearing voices network

2.   The work of Romme and Escher and the research evidence

3.   A one day training module

4.   Developing practice

The development of this manual has been informed firstly by our own work with people who hear voices, secondly by the work of the hearing voices network worldwide and thirdly by the work of Marius Romme and Sandra Escher. We are confident that on completion of this manual, participants will be much more at ease when working with people who hear voices.

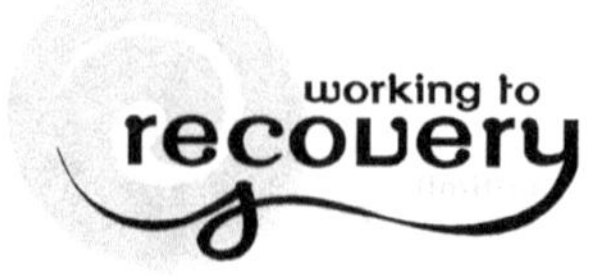

SECTION ONE
A PRACTICAL HISTORY OF THE
HEARING VOICES NETWORK

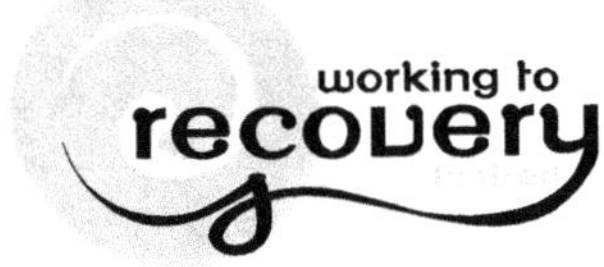

Section One: Background and potted history of the hearing voices network

A new way of thinking about hearing voices

In November 1988 Professor Romme and Sandra Escher hosted a conference in Maastricht entitled "People Who Hear Voices". The conference was held in the MECC, a prestigious National Conference Centre in Maastricht, Netherlands, and was organised jointly with Resonance (a self help organisation of people who hear voices) and the Department of Social Psychiatry at Limburg University. The conference was an opportunity for professionals to hear the direct experiences of people who hear voices, alongside current theoretical frameworks as to what the phenomenon means. It also presented a radical explanation as to the meaning of hearing voices for individuals, and ways that people could cope with this experience.

The key to this explanation was to take hearing voices out of the sickness model and such was the credibility of this approach in Holland, that the meeting was opened by the Chief Inspector for Mental Health from the Ministry of Health & Welfare for the Netherlands. The conference followed three years of work, which had presented many challenges to the current understanding of hearing voices.
When Paul Baker interviewed Marius Romme just after the conference he *(Romme)* recalled that:

"Deciding to hold a conference was not my decision, but was the decision of the Foundation Resonance. The patients felt that professionals were not accepting the voices as reality. This time a smaller number of people hearing voices and a larger number of professional people were invited. By talking and explaining their experiences to the professionals, they hoped to help enlighten people to what was actually happening, as opposed to the professionals' theory of what was happening. They were trying to bridge the gap by enabling the professionals to meet normal, healthy people who heard voices without being psychotic. These people had learnt to cope with the voices by having their own theory which acted as an anchor for them". (1)

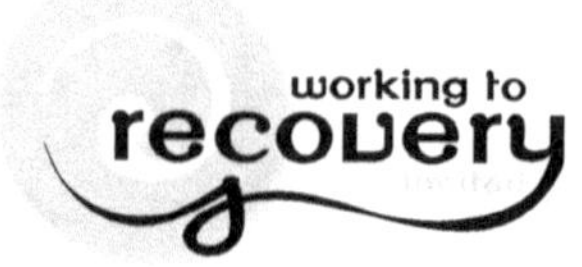

During his time in Holland Paul met Patsy Hage, a young woman who was a patient of Marius who heard voices. It was Patsy who started the whole investigation into the meaning of voices in the Netherlands. Patsy's story is a fascinating and painful one, she was hearing destructive and negative voices that gave her orders, or forbade her to do things. When Paul met her, she told him that there were times when they could dominate her completely. Patsy, who was 30 years old at the time, had already been hospitalised several times and was diagnosed as suffering from schizophrenia. She was given major tranquillisers (sometimes called neuroleptics or anti-psychotics) like many other patients who hear voices, but they had no effect on neutralising or reducing the number or the insistence of the voices she heard, as the medication is meant to do. They did, however, reduce the anxiety she felt about the existence and nature of the voices, but at the same time they also lowered her mental alertness. Patsy, understandably, found this very disturbing and was depressed by her inability to feel and think like she used to be able to. It was during this time that Patsy began to talk about suicide more often, and her psychiatrist, Marius, felt that he might be unable to prevent her from taking a path of no return. Except for one positive element in their relationship, this could have been a sad but familiar story and which has led to the death of many people diagnosed as having schizophrenia.

The positive element was that Patsy had developed her own theory about her experience of hearing voices, as many other voice hearers have and that she had the good fortune to meet a psychiatrist who was prepared to take her seriously. As Patsy explained to Marius, it was her opinion that the voices were not part of an illness neither were they hallucinations, for they had been with her since she was eight years old, appearing shortly after she had been badly burnt (subsequently it has been shown that up to 70% of voice hearers first hear voices after a major trauma). At first the voices were friendly and helpful and for a long time they caused her no problems and it was only when she was fifteen years old that the voices became unfriendly and angry. Instead, Patsy explained that for her, the voices were real, part of whom she was and although she now suffered as a result of what the voices told her, they still had meaning to her. As Patsy said to Marius: *"You believe in a God we never see or hear, so why shouldn't you believe in the voices I really do hear?"* Marius was very impressed by Patsy's point of view, for like many other psychiatrists he had always dismissed voices as being part of the delusional and hallucinatory world of the psychiatrically ill. But there was something compelling about what she had said that made sense to Marius because it was certainly the case in our society that to believe in the existence of God, in spite of the lack of any physical evidence, is acceptable and no one who believes in this is thought of as mad, yet the same acceptance is not extended to those who psychiatry regards as hallucinators.

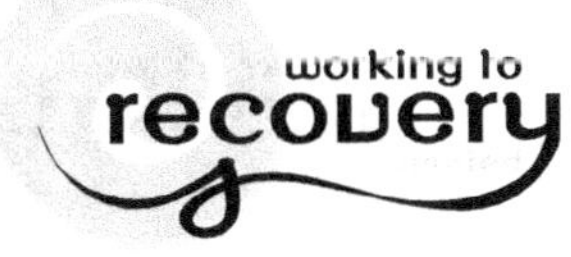

After struggling to accept this rather startling point of view for more than a year, he eventually came to believe that Patsy did really hear her voices and that they were indeed meaningful to her. For Marius this was a big step, as he was effectively walking away from the accepted mainstream medical view of what voices meant (e.g.. nothing), and on the say so of one of his patients was prepared to let go of what his own psychiatric training had taught him. Instead he took his lead from Patsy, a diagnosed schizophrenic because what she had said made more sense then any other theory he had heard. At some risk then he decided to try to do something positive with this new perspective. Thus began a journey that continues to this day, a journey that crucially has always involved voice hearers and others finding out together what this experience might mean and how it might be overcome.

Marius eventually came to think that it was possible that hearing voices could be considered to be more akin to a variation of the human mind - just as we have physical variations, for example, left handedness - and not as he previously thought a symptom of a mental disorder. So, as a scientist he decided to test the hypothesis that voices might not be part of an illness. As a consequence he invited other people who heard voices who were patients to talk about their experience and found that although they could talk about their experiences together, they could not necessarily help each other overcome the distressing feelings they had. This then did not prove much, for even if voices were "real", if they caused distress in people they still would be regarded as negative because they were causing illness. It occurred to him that because the patients had been in psychiatry for some time and clearly had other problems besides their voices and as result they might not be in a position to cope well with their experience, possibly as a result of their medication and the effects of being institutionalised as psychiatric patients

Then in an inspired and risky move, given the orthodox view of the meaning of hearing voices, Marius Romme and Patsy Hage appeared on a popular Dutch Television talk show called Vara and talked about what they had learnt about the voice hearing experience and asked for people who heard voices to phone in after the programme if they were willing to be involved in an investigation of these experiences. To their amazement over 450 people rang up, far beyond their expectations and equally surprising was the fact that 150 of those people said they were coping with their voices without assistance from psychiatry, indeed some said that on the contrary they were happy to hear their voices. These findings proved to be most important because it led to some crucial questions.

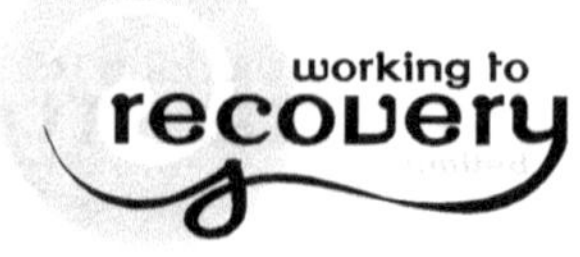

- Why was it that some people could apparently hear voices and remain healthy and others could not?

- If there was something different about the healthy voice hearers and those troubled by the experience what was it?

- If this difference could be identified could it be of any use to voice hearers troubled by their voices?

Thus Marius, Sandra and colleagues began the study of voice hearer's experiences, which continues to this day. They did two more things. In 1987 they assisted the founding of a movement of voice hearers (both within psychiatry and those who have had no contact with psychiatry), relatives, friends and professionals in Holland called WEERLANK (best translated as "Resonance") which was set up to break down the taboo of voice hearing by promoting acceptance of voices and the emancipation of voice hearers; to help break down the isolation of voice hearers and to help them cope better with their experiences. Weerlank has set up self-help groups; a telephone support network; publishes a newsletter and is actively disseminating information and guidance about voice hearing. Its aim is to encourage a change of attitude in their understanding and treatment of voices by the medical profession. Sandra Escher meanwhile, co-organises annual conferences for voice hearers and professionals and uses her journalistic skills to ensure coverage in newspapers, magazines and the electronic media with the objective of opening up discussion in society as a whole about what voices mean and to try to generate more tolerance and understanding of people who are distressed by this experience. Her particular interest is the experiences of children who hear voices and in 1993 she organised a special conference in Amsterdam for 27 children and their parents, all of whom made contact as a result of media coverage. It was held at the city zoo and the success of the event led to Sandra undertaking a research project exploring the particular experience of 80 children who hear voices, the research project was started in 1995 and was completed in 1999.

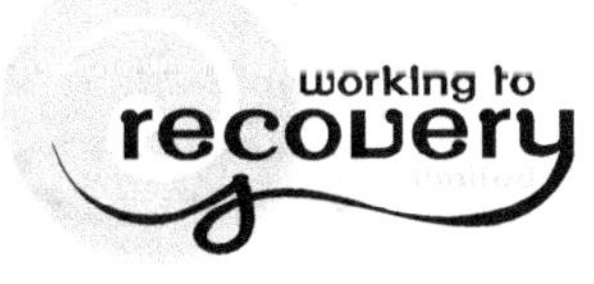

This approach has been subsequently replicated in the UK and other parts of Europe. In the UK for instance there has also been a lot of press coverage, a book published and the BBC Horizon series produced a documentary on the subject in 1995, whilst the Hearing Voices Network also runs self help groups, publishes a newsletter and holds regular conferences and meetings on the issue. Paul left the Netherlands with this challenge from Marius to develop the work in the UK:

"I ask you to try to do the same in England. Groups need to be established in each country where people can talk together about hearing voices.....it takes groups of people with the same experience to change attitudes......in America and England now, psychiatrists are following the needs of parent organisations. My goal is not changing psychiatry, not changing parents, but offering people who are hearing voices an organisation from which they can emancipate themselves. You have to organise groups, and then psychiatry follows."
(Marius Romme in interview with Paul Baker in November 1988)

He also said (I think with his tongue in his cheek) that it was possible that hearing voices by so called "normal" people was something unique to the Dutch and he was curious to discover if any British people heard them too - as it happened they did.

That was twenty-six years ago and although the task remains the same a lot of developments have occurred since then which have validated the early findings. A new way of thinking about hearing voices and even more importantly, a new way of helping people who are troubled by their voices is being developed.

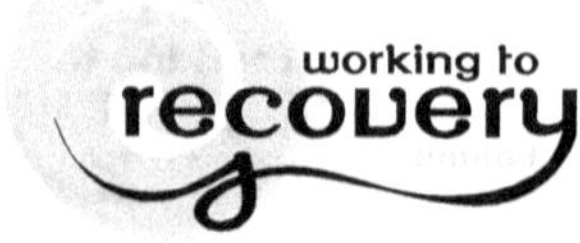

Why is redefining the experience of hearing voices so important? As you will know by now, to hear a voice that have no apparent physical cause, is usually regarded by psychiatry as an auditory hallucination, a sign of a mental illness. It is most often regarded as an important symptom of schizophrenia (although voices can also occur in manic depressive and disssociative disorders).

We all know and probably fear the stereotyped voice hearers' we sometimes see walking in the street conducting an animated conversation with themselves. There is a well worn joke about talking to yourself being the first sign of a nervous break down and it is certainly a behaviour that is likely to have the label of "mad" stamped on it - and no one really likes to think of themselves as mad. Unsurprisingly, then, hearing voices is not generally talked about because it is thought of as a socially stigmatising and unwanted experience. Romme and Escher established that the voice hearing experience had three phases; they called these the startling phase, the organisational phase and the stabilisation phase.

Most voice hearers describe the onset of the experience as being quite sudden startling and anxiety provoking and can vividly remember the precise moment they first heard a voice.

The age of the onset of the initial experience of voices varies widely as does the intensity of the startling phase, which appears to be most severe when it occurs during adolescence. The confusion seems to be less when voices are heard from an early age, or do not make an appearance until later in adulthood. (In a survey 6% heard voices before the age of six, 10% between ten and twenty and 74% after the age of twenty).

Voices are often triggered by traumatic or emotional events such as accidents, abuse, divorce, bereavement, illnesses or psychotherapy sessions.

The impact of the voices fall into two types:-

1. Some people perceive the voices as helpful and they evoke a feeling of recognition. These people feel the purpose of the voices is strengthening them and raising their self-esteem. The voices are experienced as positive and as an understandable aspect of their internal selves.

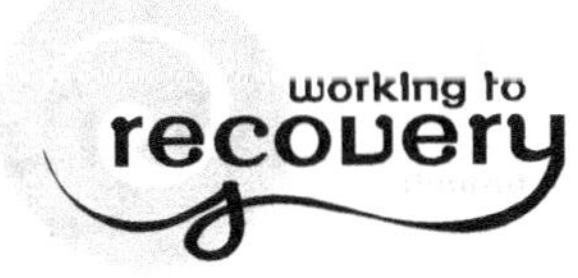

2. Others experience the voices as aggressive and negative from the very beginning. For these people the voices are hostile and are not accepted as part of themselves. They suffer from negative voices that can cause chaos in their minds, demanding so much attention that communication with the outside world is extremely difficult.

Voice hearers often become confused by their voices and want to escape from them. For some, this urge lasts only a short time (weeks or months), for others, it can be many years. However, to come to terms with the voices on any level - or – to organise them successfully, requires some form of acceptance to take place, denying the voices does not work.

During this phase, voice hearers understandably seek ways of controlling or coping with voices strategies include:

- **Ignoring the voices (through distraction)**
- **Listening to them selectively**
- **Entering into willing dialogue with them**
- **Making specific appointments with them**

Attempts at distraction and ignoring the voices rarely work, although this is a strategy many voice hearers attempt, it seems the effort involved leads to a severe restriction of life style. Unsurprisingly, initial feelings of panic and powerlessness are replaced with a period of anger at the voices this anger does not appear to be part of a useful coping strategy. The most useful strategy described by voice hearers is to select the positive voices and listen and talk only to them, and to try to understand them.

An important element in coping successfully with voices is to accept them. This appears to be related to a process of growth towards taking responsibility for one's own decisions. You have to learn to think in a positive way about yourself, your voices and your own problems.

Another strategy is to set limits and structure the contact with the voices, sometimes accompanied by rituals or repeated actions.

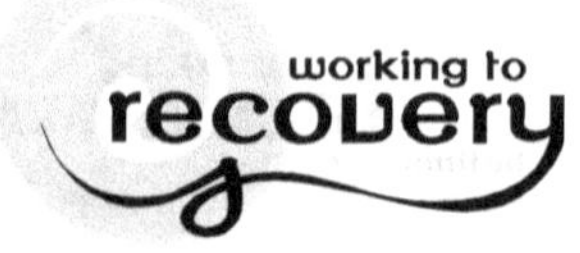

People can and do learn to cope with their voices and find a kind of equilibrium. In this state of balance, people consider the voices as part of themselves and their lives and capable of a positive influence. During this phase, the individual is able to choose between following the advice of the voices or their own ideas and can say "I hear voices and I'm happy about it".

NB: The information about the three phases of voice hearing is taken from the work of Marius Romme and Sandra Escher (see Accepting Voices)

Now discuss the following questions in light of the above information

Why was it that some people could apparently hear voices and remain healthy and others could not?

If there was something different about the healthy voice hearers and those troubled by the experience what was it?

If this difference could be identified could it be of any use to voice hearers troubled by their voices?

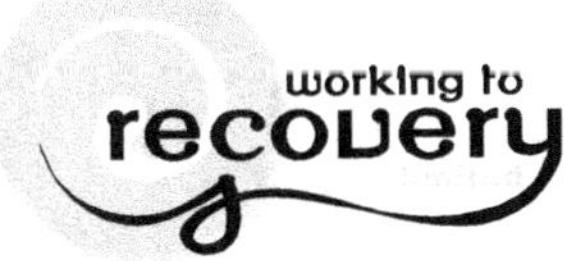

SECTION TWO
THE WORK OF ROMME & ESCHER

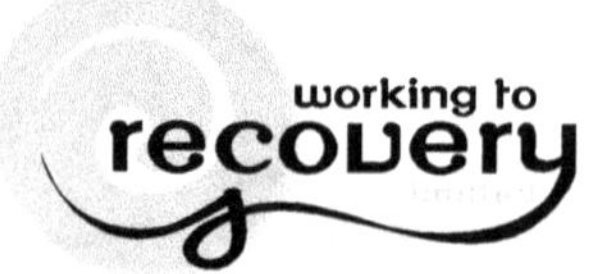

The work of Romme and Escher has been fundamental in changing how voice hearing is perceived by both professionals and voice hearers. They have pioneered much of the new ways of working with people who hear voices and developed the Maastricht interview schedule as firstly a research tool and then as way of helping the voice hearer make sense of their experience.

The problem with existing theories and treatments

Starting from the position that voice hearers are told there is no value in talking to their voices, as this is seen as entering into the delusional world of their hallucination, whilst professionals are taught not to talk to voice hearers about their voices as this is considered as a way of reinforcing the illness. Yet, at the same time voice hearers will tell you that the world of their voices are of great significance to them, apparently an impasse exists. Meanwhile, mainstream treatments for people troubled by abusive and commanding voices are as we know, limited, palliative rather than curative and involve the long-term use of powerful medicines such as major tranquilisers (neuroleptics). This treatment is known to have damaging side effects, such as weight gain, loss of vitality, a lowering of sexual libido, the flattening of emotions and a feeling of inner restlessness - it also is suspected of having longer term unwanted effects, such as damage to brain function and motor skills, an increased risk of diabetes, heart disease and cancer. Further research by Falloon and Talbot (1985) demonstrated that in only approximately 30% of patients receiving medication did the voices disappear completely and only then if taken continuously; in another 30% the voices remain in spite of taking medication, however, anxiety and chaotic thinking related to the experience is reduced; but, in the remaining 30% the medication does not influence the voices at all. Many of us have been troubled by the lack of complementary treatments and methods to assist voice hearers to cope better. In fact, this view is reinforced by the psychiatric orthodoxy that presumes that there is little the voice hearer, can do for themselves except wait for the cure for schizophrenia, (which is yet to be found and is unlikely to be) meanwhile according to this view the prognosis for many people who hear voices remains gloomy.

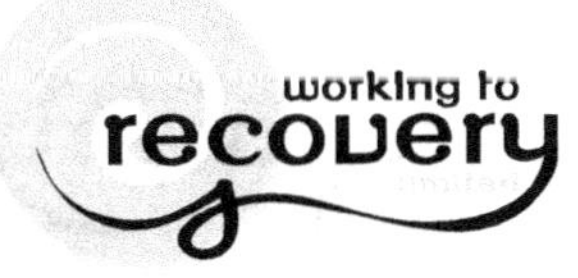

The challenge of the research to psychiatry's view of voices

There has been a small but significant number of researchers interested in the hallucinatory experiences of so called "normal people", surprisingly it began in 1889 when a man called Sidgewick was commissioned by The Society of Psychical Research to carry out interviews with a large group of ordinary people, in fact over the next three years his team of researchers interviewed 17,000 adults asking them:

"Have you ever, when believing yourself to be completely awake, had a vivid impression of seeing or being touched by a living being or inanimate object, or of hearing a voice; which impression, so far as you could discover, was not due to any external cause."

Those who responded positively were then followed up for more detail about their experience. The study found that there were a large number of voice hearers. Over a hundred years later, in a sort of follow up study to Sidgewick's, a large scale survey of 15,000 people in Baltimore, St Louis and Los Angeles carried out by A. Y Tien found that voices are heard by a substantial number regularly and continuously by 4% of the general population (in the UK, that makes for a lot of people). In the last twenty years there has been more research on the experience of voices amongst normal people, most notably by researchers: Posey and Losch, Myrtle Heery, Marius Romme and of course: A.Y. Tien, Beaven and others have confirmed that voice hearing is as commonly experienced today. These studies of groups of students (including one of medical students!), lone sailors, survivors of torture etc. have shown that as many as 55% of us have had such an experience at some time in our life (often following traumatic events such as bereavement, loss and major life changes). These people are apparently diagnosable as psychiatrically ill, yet most of them do not seek recourse to psychiatric assistance - in fact they accept their voice experience and cope with it.

The researchers, practitioners and involved voice hearers believe it is mistaken to regard voice hearing as part of a psychopathic disease syndrome. Rather, they consider it to be more akin to a variation in human experience - if you like, a faculty or differentiation - something like homosexuality, and that it is definitely not open to cure. This view may sound radical, but is based on sound, quality research involving questionnaires and interviews conducted with many voice hearers, both within and outside of psychiatry. What was found, was most surprising, voice hearers cope with their voices (or conversely don't), not because of the content of the voice experience (which can be either abusive and devaluing or guiding

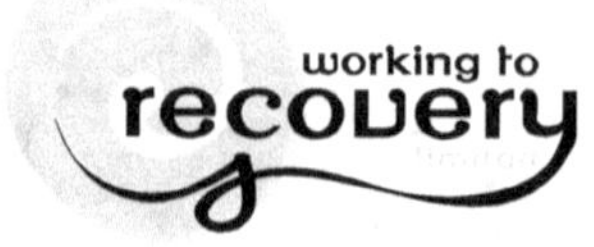

and inspiring - or both) but because of the nature of the relationship with the voices. Bottom line, this means that if you believe the voices to be in control you can't cope - if you believe you are stronger then the voices are, you can.

As a result of these findings it is no longer a sustainable position to think of voices as part of a disease syndrome, such as schizophrenia, instead hearing voices can be regarded as a meaningful, real (although sometimes painful, fearful and overwhelming) event, that speak to the person in a metaphorical way about their lives, emotions and environment. For instance, people experiencing distress as a consequence of abusive or commanding voices can often recognise their voices as those of their actual abusers and the voices have the effect of attacking their sense of self-esteem and worth. It should not be forgotten however, that some people experience helpful and guiding voices, also arising from times of trauma and stress.

Having discovered these kinds of relationships psychiatrists and psychologists in the UK and the Netherlands are developing techniques to assist voice hearers focus on their experience and get to know their voices better. This flies in the face of psychiatric and psychological orthodoxies that assume that such psychopathological symptoms are not open to insight and talking treatments and instead would attempt to distract patients with such symptoms from their voices. This turns out not only to be bad advice, but actually counterproductive, as such approaches disempower the voice hearer by denying to them their real experience and disarming them from taking on the voices and standing up for themselves. The new approach requires the voice hearer to make space for the voices, to listen but not to necessarily follow, to engage, but in their own time and space - essentially to learn how to control them in their own terms, according to their own beliefs and explanatory framework. This acceptance of the voices is crucial to growth and resolution, voice hearers who have learnt these techniques can now say: "I hear voices, they are part of me and I am glad they are"

Focusing on the meaning of voices

It became evident that it was important to explore the relationship between the hearing of voices and the life history of the voice hearer in order to see if it was possible to help them to solve their emotional and other problems. This approach emphasises the importance of understanding what the voices were saying to the voice hearer and required them to focus their attention on the voices as a way of finding a resolution to the difficulties they caused. In doing so, however, it was considered very important to

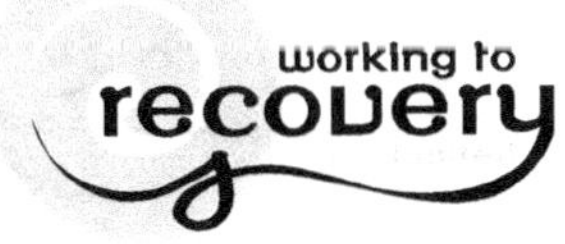

develop a way of working that was cooperative and based on mutual trust; as a result the following features of the voice hearing experience have been investigated by Professor Romme, Sandra Escher and the Maastricht team:

- **The identity of the voices**

- **The characteristics of their communication with the person; the way of talking**
  - The age of the voices
  - What they have to say?

- **What triggers the appearance of the voices?**

- **What important changes in the life of the voice hearer were related to the appearance of the voices?**

- **Characteristics of the voice hearer's upbringing and any special experiences that occurred in childhood**

As a result of this research, which was carried out using questionnaires and one to one interviews the following important information was found out about the triggering of voices: they often arise when experiencing certain threatening or overwhelming emotions such as insecurity, fear, aggression, ones own sexual feelings, the sexual feelings of others, losing control; or when confronted by certain situations (feeling out of control or losing control) such as new situations, unexpected situations, the company of new people, situations that create stress, the feelings of others in the same room, fatigue etc.

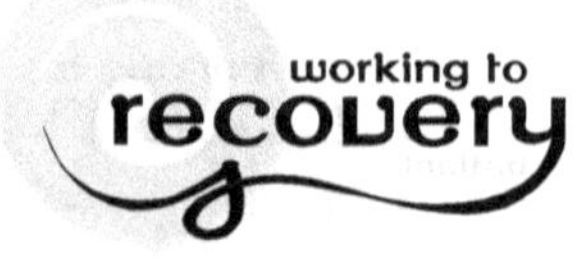

The research also showed it is very important to recognise that the voices know the person who hears them very well and that they always say things that are especially relevant to them and that are related to their problems. The voices usually refer to unsolved problems in daily life and/or emotions related to a trauma that has not yet been resolved, or to unrealised hopes and aspirations that, in some cases, are impossible to realise. Therefore in working with a voice hearer it is not valid to reject the voices instead, it is more appropriate to stimulate the curiosity of the voice hearer about what the voices are saying. As long as the voice hearer is only able to react to the voices in an emotional way, they are disempowered by the voices and it is therefore difficult to stimulate their curiosity. This process is difficult to accomplish and over the last five years the Maastricht team have been exploring techniques that appeal to people hearing voices. This exploration was also conducted in cooperation with people hearing voices and as a result the following constructive techniques used by people hearing voices to improve their coping skills: Give the voices a specific time; talk back to the voices; set limits; write down what they say; find someone with whom you can talk about your voices

In the last seventeen years, especially in England, university psychologically departments have been trying out techniques used in cognitive therapy, to see if they are of assistance to voice hearers. This has proved to be quite a promising development. Besides techniques used generally in anxiety management, a more specific method has been developed to explore the relationship between the voices and the person's life situation. This technique is known as focusing and has been developed by the psychologists Gillian Haddock and Richard Bentall, focusing examines the characteristics of the voices, the kind of relationship that exists between the voices and the person who hears them and explores the possibility of changing these relationships. The experience of the workers in the UK and the Netherlands is that if the total attention in therapy is focused on treating the "illness" rather then the problems in daily life, as expressed by the voices will not be solved. The main objective is not only to influence the methods used in coping with the voices but also to change the manner in which the person copes with their daily life problems and emotions. Thereby, giving them more control over the negative and abusive content of the voice experience.

By asking questions about coping strategies that voice hearers have evolved for themselves in dealing with their voices can help determine how active or passive the voice hearer is in relationship with the voices. It is often the case that voice hearers are unaware that there maybe other more effective ways then the ones they employ. By learning more about coping strategies, it has been possible to determine which ones appear to be the most effective.

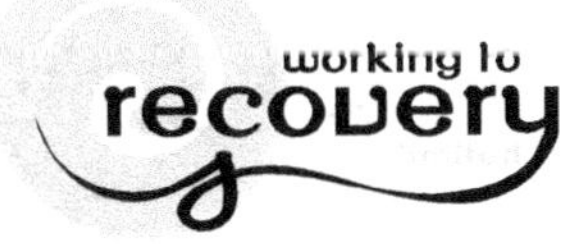

Coping Strategies

There have been three strategies identified to date all of them require as a first step, an acceptance of the voices existence:

1. Cognitive Strategies: These include the following: ignoring the voices, listening to them, listening selectively, sending the voices away, and maintaining a discussion with them. Cognitive strategies do offer a greater degree of control over the voices; whilst ignoring the voices is still to be in flight from the voices; listening can help control the fear of voices even if it remains a passive relationship; Listening selectively, however is more active and the research shows that most non-patient voice hearers use this method; sending the voices away is an active strategy, but not as effective as maintaining discussion, which means that the voice hearer is able to answer "yes" or "no" to the voices or conversely to ask questions of the voices themselves.

2. Behavioural Strategies: These include the following: distraction (e.g. using personal stereos), reaching agreement re. times to talk with the voices, keeping a diary. Behavioural coping strategies again have varying degrees of effectiveness; distraction is mainly a flight mechanism and useful mainly for short term relief. Reaching an agreement with the voices to provide a way of giving some order to the experience; keeping a diary as means of getting more insight into the meaning of the voices, their frequency and their vocabulary or talking to a therapist about them is more active and effective.

3. Physiological: These include the following: alcohol, drugs etc., medication, relaxation exercises, tai chi, diet. The use of alcohol and recreational drugs is mostly a flight mechanism, that few people say they use; the use of medication has the effect of accepting a subordinate relationship to the voices; whilst relaxation exercise and dietary techniques offer a means of gaining control through ordering the experience.

When the team asked which methods voice hearers, who were patients, used most and which they thought were most effective, they found that on the whole they were very limited in what they used and on the whole they were not effective and further they were not aware that there were other methods they could use. Voice hearers who had never been patients, however, were using a much wider range of the effective techniques and were benefiting from them. This shows that there is some hope that these methods can be taught and utilised by people who are distressed by their voices and indeed this is proving to be the case, but also is an indictment against the existing psychiatric treatments and methods.

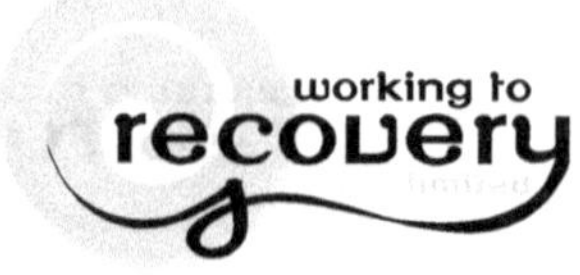

The story behind these developments is a powerful indictment of the importance of professionals listening and working in partnership with the people who experience voice hearing. Rather then making assumptions, they drew lessons from the experts, the voice hearers themselves.

For mental health workers these steps may demand a considerable enlargement of clinical perspective, and a broadening of the generally accepted theories within the profession. We have found that mental health teams across the world with the support of Working to Recovery, Intervoice, the Maastricht team and the growing hearing voices networks. This work is being complimented by the provision of training the development of self- help groups, to conclude it seems appropriate to quote Marius Romme:

"What this research shows us is that we must accept that the voices exist. We must also accept that we cannot change the voices. They are not curable, just as you cannot cure left-handedness or dyslexia - human variations are not open to cure - only to coping. Therefore to assist people to cope, we should not give them therapy that does not work. We should let people decide for themselves what helps or not. It takes time for people to accept that hearing voices is something that belongs to them." Marius Romme

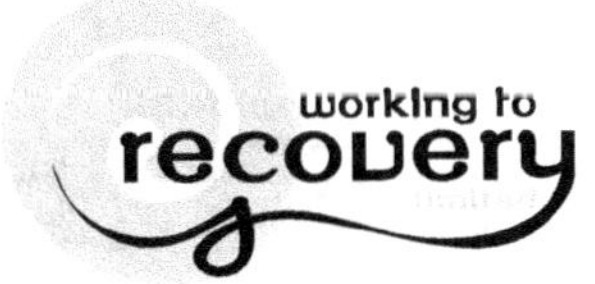

Research conclusions:

The research and practice has shown the following:

(i)   Hearing voices is neither a disease entity, nor does it refer to a specific psychiatric disorder;

(ii)   For mental health workers it is less of significance to know if someone hears voices (as in a "so called" indicator for schizophrenia) than in understanding if the voices have any detrimental effects on the persons' quality of life;

(iii)   Because of the presence of voice hearing in healthy people, voices can only be considered to sign of a mental health problem when there are other evident symptoms;

(iv)   In general, assistance from psychiatric and other psychotherapeutic help is only required if the voices are subjectively experienced as being negative by the voice hearer;

(v)   Because the voices have a meaning, are real to the person and have metaphoric significance, it is clearly the case, that, if the voices are causing problems then talking therapies are a valid, if not vital intervention (something that is generally not recognised within traditional psychiatry for so called psychopathological conditions). Specifically, the use of the following techniques is proving effective:

Anxiety management to give more control; focusing in order to give more control; promoting people's social opportunities and self esteem in order to assist them develop their capacity to live in society.

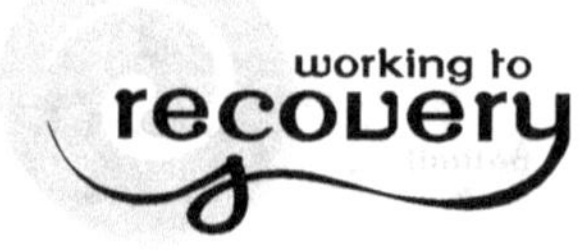

SECTION THREE
A ONE DAY VOICES WORKSHOP

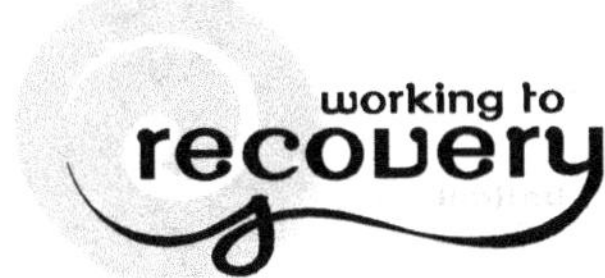

This one-day workshop is designed to introduce workers, carers and users to new ways of working with those who hear voices. It is based on workshops that we have delivered since 1991. The aim of the workshop is to provide people with an alternative way of thinking from that of the medical model. A one-day workshop cannot give people the skills they require to work with everyone who hears voices and it has never been our intention to do this. What it can do, however is to give workers, carers and users an opportunity to explore the world of voices from different perspectives.

Many workers are already working with voice hearers in different ways, many of them have told us it feels more natural to work in these ways and more importantly many have told us that their clients have benefited from these ways of working. In the mid 1990s some of us started talking about the possibility of recovery-based programmes as opposed to maintenance based work. In 1998 however the UK Government made it clear that they were about to legitimise a policy of social control based on compliance with medication rather than on what was best for each individual. Our belief is that this has made it more difficult for workers to engage with clients in a positive way. This shift in policy makes it more important that we work with those who hear voices in ways, which do not alienate them further.

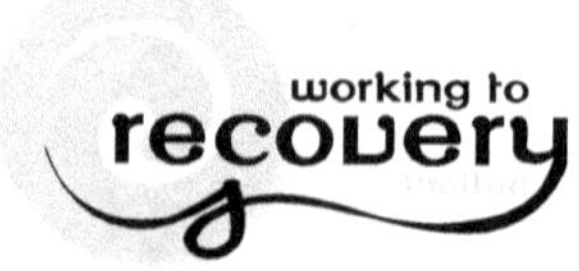

(1)   The voice hearing experience:

This session includes a case study, a simulation exercise and group discussion

(2)   A bad career move:

This session is based on a DVD, which explores a journey through psychosis as perceived by the voice hearer. The DVD is 1 hour long and is in two sections, the first section focuses on the persons' recollections of the system whilst the second section looks at the relationship between the voices and the person's life history. This is followed by a discussion in the group, which should be based on their experiences of working with voice hearers

(3)   Frames of Reference and Voice profiling:

This session uses as its main aids the workbook **"Working With Voices 2, Victim to Victor" (Coleman & Smith 2005 P & P Press)** The main aim of this part of the day is to explore some of the frames of reference that voice hearers have for their voices and how to profile voices in a way which allows both the worker and the voice hearer to make sense of the voices

(4)   Practical ways of working with voices:

This session will look at one case study of a voice hearer, their belief system, and how they were able to resolve their problem with voices within their belief system. Trainees will also have an opportunity to discuss how they can adapt this way of working with their clients

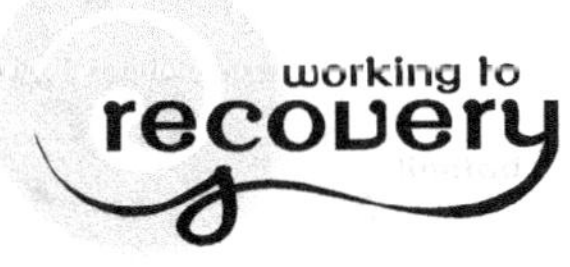

The voice hearing experience

Introduce yourself to the group, take your time approximately fifteen minutes tell the group about your background, the fact you have been through this course yourself and what you will be expecting from them for the duration of the course. Ask if they have any questions or fears about the course and try to deal with any that arise. Do not worry if you cannot, simply tell the person you will get back to them at the next session.

You are now ready to start

A case study. (**Read only the part in green italics to the group**)

CASE STUDY

The subject is male about 30 years of age, he wanders off and stops looking after himself. Then he starts to hear voices - there are two voices one is the voice of God the other is the voice of the devil. He is told that he can jump from high places and not harm himself. He is also told that he can own half the world if he surrenders to the voice. The man comes through this experience unscathed then goes into a city enters a big civic building trashes the place and throws people about.

The question for the group is: What would our society do with this man?

The following is the normal response that groups give to the above question allow your group to discuss the question. Do not allow then to get politically correct with statements such as "We would assess the man first" as this frequently does not happen.

Acting in the way that he is he clearly represents a danger to himself and to other people. His delusional thoughts and hallucinations are controlling his actions and as a result he would probably be arrested, be seen by a police surgeon and taken to the local psychiatric hospital, where if he did not accept being admitted voluntarily he would be sectioned and then he would be treated again against his will if need be. The psychiatrist would then try all sorts of combinations of drugs to eliminate the voices, the view of all the service providers will be a simple one ... get the person ... well and make him better.

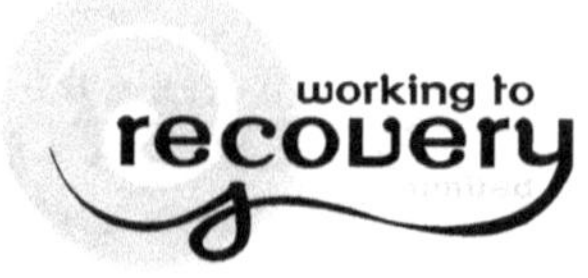

Once you have teased out the above scenario tell the group what actually happened in this case, for it is a real case, the voice hearer was crucified and we now call him the Son of God or Jesus.

Remember, we are told in the bible how Jesus wanders off into the desert, starts hearing not only his father's voice, but also the voice of Lucifer. He is told that if he jumps from the top of the cliff, he will not be dashed on the rocks, or if he follows Lucifer he will be given half his kingdom to rule. Later, Christ goes to the temple where he finds the moneylenders plying their trade upon which Christ threw tables all over the place and threw the money lenders out of the temple. So right at the very beginning of this session we can see that just describing a set of symptoms and behaviour patterns can lead us to make conclusions that are false. Most of us would have sectioned the Son of God and probably called him a psychotic or even schizophrenic.

Let the group discuss their response, when they have finished their discussion ask how many of them have heard voices ay least once in their lives. Normally when you ask this question very few participants will admit to hearing voices, your role at this point is to ask other questions that will enable them to explore this idea. These questions can include:

- How many of you just as you are falling asleep or just wakening up have heard someone shout your name looked around and found no one there?

- How many of you have heard music with no possible source?

- How many of you have heard your name called when walking down the street and could not see anyone?

- How many of you have heard what has been called their conscience especially when they were younger and did something wrong?

By this point most of the group will admit to having an experience where they have heard something. From this fact it is possible to assert that hearing things or voices is not the problem rather it is what is done with the experience or how we might respond to the experience that may become a problem. Now tell the group they are about to experience negative voices.

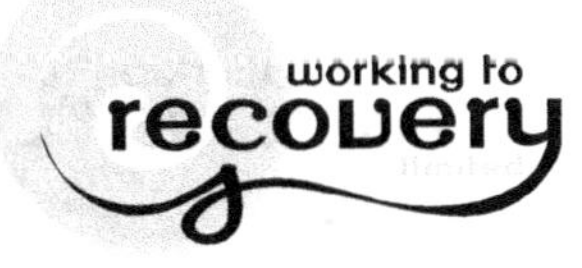

Split the group into threes, two facing each other and having a conversation and one to be a voice. The person who is being the voice should get up close to the ear of one of the people having the conversation and say nasty things into the persons ear they should continue to say nasty things for a minute or so, then the participants should change places until everyone has been both the voice and the voice hearer.

Once everyone has taken part in the exercise bring the group back together and ask them if this was to happen to them outside of an exercise situation what would the consequences ensure you use the word consequences are for them. Use a flip chart to record answers, record answers to each question as you go along.

1.   *Firstly ask them how they would feel?*
2.   *Secondly ask them what would happen to their thinking.*
3.   *Thirdly what would happen to their speech?*
4.   *Fourthly what would happen to their job, relationships and what state would their house be in?*
5.   *Fifthly ask them if they would believe the voices. If they say they would believe the voices, ask them if they would believe the voices if they said they were from outer space and coming to take them away?*

When you get the answer yes ask them what this would be classed as? The answer you are looking for is a delusion.

The next question is to ask them what they would do about it? When it appears that no more answers are forthcoming give them one final chance to add anything else to the list.
Ask the group where they might find a list like this? They should give answers such as: in the patients notes both medical and nursing notes, psychiatric text books, reports and the answer we are looking for diagnostic manuals such as the Diagnostic Statistical Manual (DSM) or the International classification of diagnosis (ICD10). Then ask the group what they would be listed as? The answer is symptoms now ask the groups Symptoms of what? The answer is of course schizophrenia.

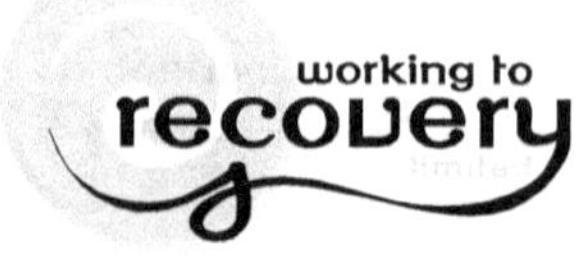

You should then point out to the group that many of these symptoms are to be found in other psychotic conditions, such as, manic depression, dissociative disorders, some forms of depression and affective disorders.

There is one major question that you should ask at this point and that is are the answers on the list are secondary symptoms of a disease process called schizophrenia or are they the consequences of the event of hearing voices. Ask the group to think about this but at this point there is no need to come up with an answer.

Ask the group to spend some time discussing the following questions.

What are their fears about the effect that voices will have on clients?
This discussion can go in many directions but at some point one member of the group will raise the most common fear that of a voice hearer obeying their voices and either harming themselves or another.

When this happens find the biggest and the smallest person in the group ask them to come and join you get them to face each other and ask the biggest person to clench their fists and then tell them to hit the other person in the face as hard as they can. When they refuse or only pretend to hit the person tell them again to hit the person for real be insistent and keep on going at them for a minute or so. Thank both of them and ask the one who was asked to do the hitting why they did not hit the person. Undoubtedly they will give you many replies in the end ask them if they made a choice the answer should be yes.

Put up overhead 1 "people who hear voices make choices"

Ask the group (by a show of hands) how many of them are working with people whose voices tell them on a regular basis perhaps even daily to kill themselves; then ask them again how many of them are still alive.

Ask the group to discuss the significance of this. Try to steer the discussion in the direction of personal responsibility.

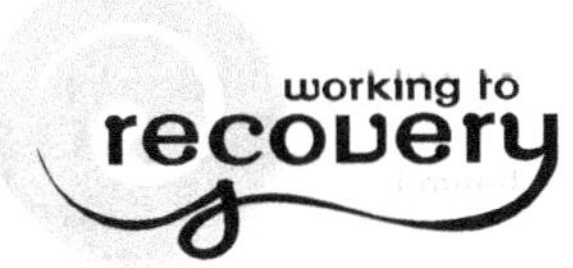

Understanding the relationship between voices and a persons' life history

Before you begin this session ask if there are any points from the morning session, if there are, allow the group to discuss them for no more than 15 minutes.

Begin this session by telling the group that you will be playing a DVD, which will sketch one person's journey through psychosis. Advise them to make notes, as the DVD will be discussed by the group when it is ended. Start the DVD.

When the DVD has ended ask the group for their initial reactions, do not worry about what is discussed at this stage just let them vent their responses to the tape.

When they have done this it is time to start a structured discussion about some of the issues.
Ask them if they have voice hearing clients who have went through similar life events such as abuse.

Discuss this if the response is no, ask them if they have ever broached the subject with their clients. If the response is yes then ask them if they think there is a relationship between the abuse and the voices. This could be that they hear the voice of their abuser.

Discuss with the group the following questions:

- Can this type of trauma be a cause of a person's voices?

- If we accept that trauma can cause voices how can we best work with the voice hearer?

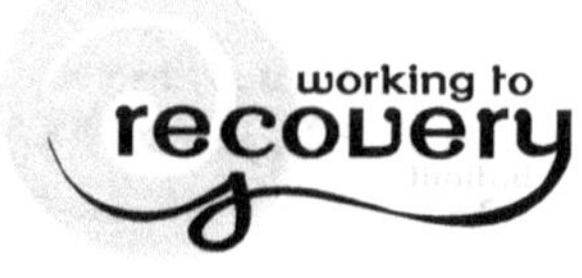

Understanding Voices

It is important that we create a safe environment in which to explore the voice hearer's experience. In order to achieve this, practitioners should take a lot of time when using these tools. This will also help create the necessary relationship for effective outcome working.

Understanding the voices that people hear requires that we develop good ways of gathering information that will enable both the worker and the voice hearer to make sense of the experience. This session will explore tools we can use to gather this information. This will include exploring the following:

1. The onset of voices

2. I've just heard voices checklist

3. The life story

4. Voice profiling

(1) The onset of voices.

When working with a voice hearer it is important that we find out as much as possible about the first voice hearing experience. There are a number of reasons for this, the main one being that the first experience can often give us clues as to the context in which, the first voice hearing experience happened. Finding the context can also help us understand triggers that make the voice experience more intense for the voice hearer.

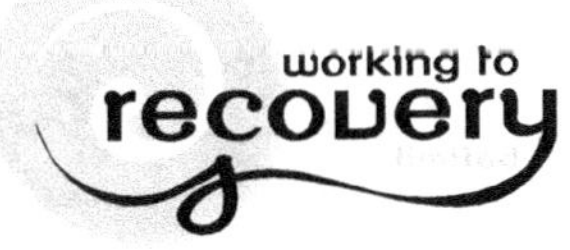

When the voice hearing experience begins there can be a multitude of responses. The very first reaction is at an emotional level whether this is positive or negative. It is not surprising that such a personal experience involves what can be the extremes of emotion. Romme and Escher describe the onset of voices as the startling phase. *The first time I heard a voice I was sitting at my desk waiting for some information from the computer when a voice behind me said "you've done that wrong". I looked around thinking it was my secretary but there was no one there. My first feeling was fear. My response was to go to the bar and get drunk.*

It is important that the client can look back to their first experience of voices. The client should write a description of their first experience of hearing voices. Include everything they can remember, it's alright to be honest. They don't have to share this with anyone they do not want to. This can be a stressful thing to do, but they should write as much as they can, even if it doesn't seem important now. Many people have told us how just writing these things down make them feel better about them.

Another tool that is useful is the "I have just heard voices checklist"-as shown on next page. This tool can be given to the client and filled in each day for ten days. Analysing what has been written may well help both the worker and the voice hearer gain further insight into the context in which the voices are being heard. *Give each participant a copy of each tool and discuss how the tools might be useful when working with voice hearers. Note the importance to both the client and the worker. Ensure that participants are okay about using the tools.*

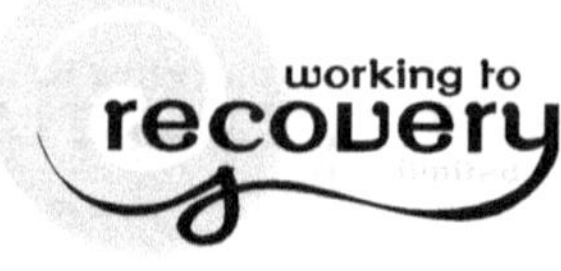

Now complete these next two pages each time you hear voices for the next 10 days at least. Feel free to photocopy these two pages.

Date ....   Time spent with voices ....

Time ....   Voluntary time with voices ....

Please be as honest as possible as this checklist is to help you identify the voices, and any things which occur that can help you to identify when the voices communicate with you, and to develop ways of predicting and organising your life to accommodate the voices.

The voices I heard were:-

1...   4...

2...   5...

3...   6...

The voices said

....

....

....

They were talking about

....

....

....

I Felt

....

....

....

I Was at (Place)

....

....

....

working to
recovery

I Was with (Company)

....

....

....

I was doing

....

....

....

The place was (Noisy, quiet, people talking)

....

....

....

I had been thinking about

....

....

....

Please answer yes or no

My state of consciousness was altered   ____

My Vision was heightened/altered   ____

I felt Paranoid   ____

I felt out of control   ____

I felt powerful   ____

My explanation for the voices is

....

....

Please add any other information that will help you develop your work either alone or with people.

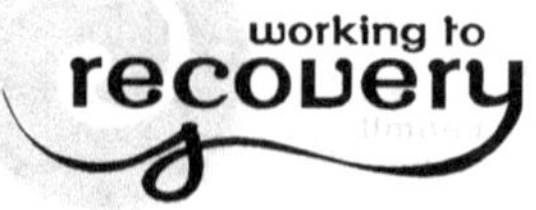

Sandra Escher has expressed on many occasions her belief that one of the most important things that a voice hearer can do is to write what she calls their ego document. An ego document is a person's life story written by them self and more importantly, for them self. **The writing of their life history is the single most important thing a voice hearer can do for themselves.** Through writing their life story in their style they can bring out what is important to them. It is an opportunity to move away from how others view their life and what has happened to them in it. We all have a story to tell about our lives, no two of which are the same. It is important that voice hearers, start to see them self as an individual rooted in society and not as a patient rooted in psychiatry. We should ask the client to write down, their own life story in a condensed form. You should ask the voice-hearer to write down in their own language and keep it simple. Tell them not to try to analyse as they are writing; just be factual. Remember, this is for them, they need never show the contents to anyone if they do want to.

Romme and Escher's' research revealed many things but one of the most important was that 70% of those they interviewed started hearing voices after what Romme and Escher called a traumatic life event. These events included death of a loved one, (normally violent e.g.. suicide or murder or accident) leaving home for the first time, abuse be it sexual, physical or emotional and being involved in a major disaster are but a few of the life experiences that voice hearers disclosed in their interviews with Romme and Escher.

When the person has finished writing their life story get them to look back at it, especially at the critical events, ask them the following; how are these things related to why they now hear voices, did it change their relationship, did it cause the voices to come, did it give them more power, do they abuse them because of it? With the critical events it helps to understand the importance of these events in their life, and how do they contribute to the person they are.

Many people relate their voices to traumatic life events (anywhere from 25-95%), however it is helpful to understand why this is so. For example many people tell of childhood sexual abuse being important or witnessing a trauma, what we are interested in is how this has affected them, for instance does the voice blame them, do they feel guilty or ashamed has it affected their ability to trust others etc. We call this creating an Ego document, you simply look at the life events that they may have listed in their life history and ask, why are these events important? For example why my father's death is so important,

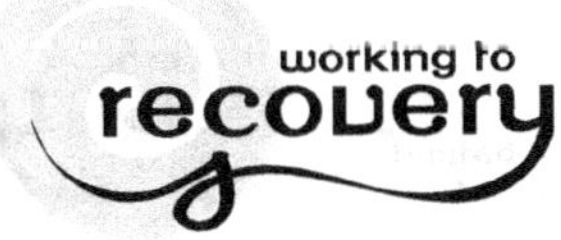

was it because I never said goodbye, was it because I wanted him to see the person I have become, was it because I feel responsible for his death or his feelings when he died?

Ask the participants to write down the three major events that have shaped their lives until now. Tell them they will not need to share these events with anyone else. When they have finished ask them if they had to share these events with the whole group how many of them would change the three? Spend sometime discussing this and relating it to the clients they know.

Voice Profiling

Voice profiling is one tool that can be used when working with voice hearers. This tool is useful in helping the voice hearer understand the characteristics' of their voices. It has become clear through the work of people like Romme and Escher that for many voice hearers their voices have clearly defined personalities that can be broken down in such a way that voice hearers are better able to understand them.

It is important when using voice profiling to start with simple questions such as how many voices do they hear? There is no point in starting with questions about the power relationship between the voice hearer and individual voices.

When the person has finished their voice profile and the other exercises the information can be used to develop some ideas around the reason they hear voices and this in turn can be used to develop ways of working with the person's voices. *Trainees will be using the voice profiling material in the last session around case working.*

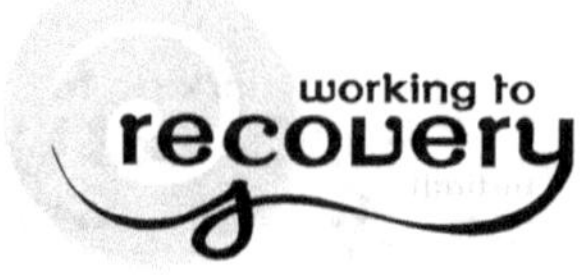

When answering the following questions take your time and think through your answer Feel free to make more comments on the page marked notes at the end of the questions. Remember you do not need to show this to anyone if you do not want to.

How many voices do you hear? ....

How many of your voices are male? ....

How many of your voices are female? ....

Are any of your voices positive?   YES   NO   SOMETIMES

If yes or sometimes how many? ....

Are any of your voices negative?   YES   NO   SOMETIMES

If yes or sometimes how many? ....

Are any of your voices advisory?   YES   NO   SOMETIMES

If yes or sometimes how many? ....

Are any of your voices commanding?   YES   NO   SOMETIMES

If yes or sometimes how many? ....

Are any of your voices abusive?   YES   NO   SOMETIMES

If yes or sometimes how many? ....

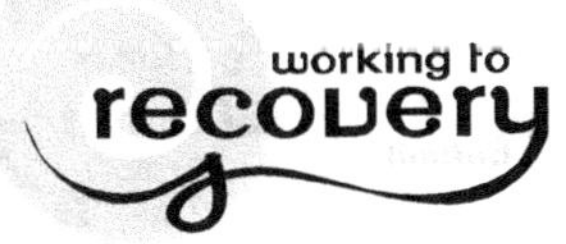

If you know the names or if you have given names to any of your voices, then list those below please feel free to comment on your voices here.

Response

....

....

....

....

....

....

....

....

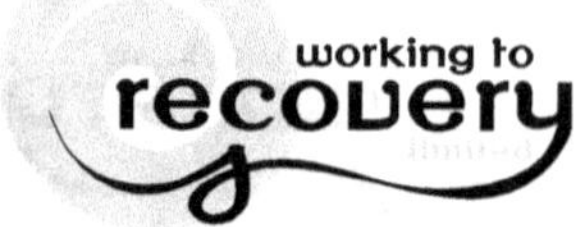

Now, to start to identify your voices and to record them so that you can begin to establish who the voices are, when you hear them, and any other relevant details. Please photocopy this list on the next two pages and fill one each time you hear the voice(s). Try to complete it as soon as possible afterwards and try to carry on your normal life whilst doing this. Do not listen for the voices any more than you normally do.

From the questions you have just answered and the voices checklist you have completed it is possible to build up a voices profile for each voice. Below you will find descriptions of three of the voices that Ron Coleman hears, not as he hears them now, but how he heard them in the early days. The three voices are called Priest who was Ron's' abuser Annabelle who was his partner who died and Neil, a close friend who also died. One of the things you should notice is the difference in personalities between the voices.

Name	Male/Female	Pos/Neg	Advisory/Command	Abusive
Priest	Male	Negative	Negative	Yes
Annabelle	Female	Both	Both	Both
Neil	Male	Positive	Advisory	Abusive

Using the rest of this sheet do the same for the voices of someone you know or your own if you hear voices. If you cannot name all the voices you may find it useful to describe them in some way e.g., they/you may think the voice reminds them of a teacher so call it Teacher, or you may think a voice is a demon so call it Demon.

Name	Male/Female	Pos/Neg	Advisory/Command	Abusive

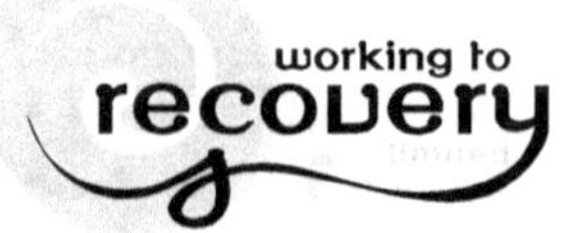

Working with Voices Practice

Use the following case study to help participants

Case Study Jenny

The first thing Jenny did was to tell her life story, which in a very shortened version went like this; when Jenny was a child she lived with her mum who was divorced from her father and she had no contact with her dad. Her mother met a new man who Jenny said was okay at first, her mother married the new man and Jenny got herself a step-dad. Although everything was good at the beginning, it was not long before her new step-dad took an interest in jenny not as a daughter but as an object that he could abuse. Jenny was abused by her step-dad for about two years before she finally told her grandmother what was happening to her. The grandmother told Jenny's mother what was going on but her mother refused to believe it, finally in frustration grandmother took jenny to live with her and brought Jenny up. Her grandmother did not go to the authorities for fear that she too would lose Jenny, Jenny was also very clear that she did not fault her grandmother for this, indeed jenny felt her grandmother had done a good job in bringing her up. Jenny married when she was in her late teens and divorced in her mid-twenties she had two children during her marriage. Her grandmother died when she was twenty-two and she felt very alone since she did not talk to her mother who was still married to Jenny's abuser.

Jenny had started hearing an occasional voice when she was in her late teens but thought nothing of it. During the break-up of her marriage her voices had got much worse and she started hearing very negative voices, it was at this time that she came to the attention of the psychiatric services. She was eventually given a diagnosis of paranoid schizophrenia and put on various neuroleptics none of which relieved the voices. She was prone to self-harming and spent a lot of her hospital admissions being detained on sections of the mental health act. She had finally managed to bring her self-harm under control though she had not stopped completely, she had got this far through membership of a self-help group.

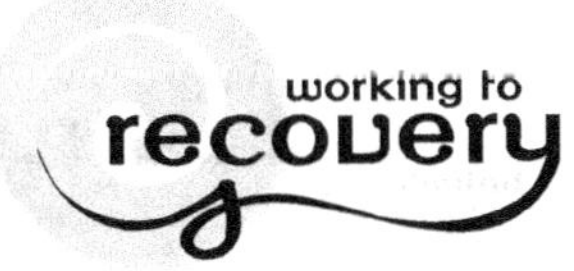

Jenny identified four voices,

Ask the group who they think the voices are as you work through the next section you should put this on a flipchart in the form of a voice profile

The first was male very negative, always abusive and commanding. This voice would tell her that it was her fault that she deserved everything that happened to her and that she was a slut. This voice she knew was the voice of her stepfather (her abuser). The second voice was in every way a contrast to the first voice it was female very positive, never abusive, it was advisory and everything it said was soothing and helpful. This voice would say that things would be okay that she (the voice) would protect Jenny. Jenny knew this to be the voice of her grandmother. The third voice was the voice of a female child who would do nothing but scream all the time. In one way this was the most difficult voice for Jenny in that it never made any sense. It was only after some time that Jenny identified the voice as the voice of herself when she was being abused. The final voice was a male voice that was a mixture of everything, it was both positive and negative, abusive and non-abusive, advisory and commanding indeed so much so we called it her neutral voice and she knew it to be the voice of her ex-husband.

Once we had a life history and a voice profile Jenny then related her voices to her life history and decided that her real problem was not the voices but the fact that she had been sexually abused and that this issue had never been properly resolved.

Before we could go any further with the voices work Jenny had to carry out one of the most difficult and lonely tasks that anyone who has been abused has to do, that is she had to find herself innocent of any fault within the abuse. This is something that everyone who has been abused has to come to terms with at some point if recovery is going to become a reality. The voice of the abuser told Jenny that it was her fault that the abuse happened and like many people who hear the voice of their abuser or abusers Jenny was inclined to believe that she did play some part in leading him on.

It did not matter that I like many others told Jenny that she was the victim in this situation what mattered is what Jenny thought was the facts. Jenny had to put herself on trial and in order to do this she had to go through the experience again and again from every conceivable angle until she could say with real conviction I am innocent. This is no easy task and anyone who has done it will tell you that not only is it painful it is also exhausting and often initially it makes the voices worse. Once this was done Jenny

and I discussed how best to work with the voices, her desire was to get rid of the voices though she knew that at best she would probably only succeed in developing coping strategies that would allow her to get on with her life.

We decided that the best way forward was to enter into dialogue with her voices and that we would do this with one voice at a time. In other words we would do what most professionals believe we should never do, that is actively engage with the voices.

Ask the group which voice they would start with. The answer should be the grandmother as she is the most positive voice.

The first attempt was almost a complete disaster, with hindsight it was my fault as I underestimated the resistance that I would encounter from the voice of the grandmother. I started by asking Jenny if she would ask her grandmother if she would talk to me. Jenny's reply astonished me, at the time she (her grandmother) wanted to know why she should talk to me and why I wanted to help Jenny. It took three meetings before the grandmother would stop asking questions as to my motives and start talking about how we might help Jenny. (After the whole process was over Jenny and I concluded that the questions her grandmother's voice was asking were in actual fact related to Jenny's own fears about the journey we were starting) After the initial breakthrough grandmother agreed to help Jenny and I deal with the voice of the stepfather. We then decided that the next voice to approach was that of her ex-husband, this was a complete and utter waste of time the voice played games with us for weeks on end before we finally decided that there would be no help for Jenny from this voice. (We came to the conclusion from this experience with the voice of the ex-husband that some voices have very little or no significance when you are working through the voice hearing experience, indeed that some voices are nothing more than red herrings)

We then turned our attention to the child voice and to our horror found that not only would the child not engage in any way with me it would not engage in any way with Jenny either. We spent many hours trying to forge a relationship with the child to no avail. Eventually we turned to the grandmother for help and asked her to negotiate with Jenny the child, the grandmother agreed and she slowly managed to get Jenny the child to talk to us but initially only through her (the grandmother). Over time Jenny the child stopped screaming and did start to talk to us, she agreed that it was her that had to confront the abuser and we spent many hours preparing Jenny the child for this confrontation. (We had in effect forgotten

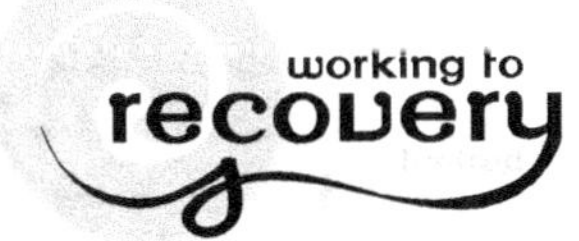

one of the rules of working with voices, which was to play to your strengths. We had started the process by enlisting the aid of the grandmother and then once getting it we had essentially left her out of the process. She was to be the key to Jenny the child as a voice as she had been the ally of Jenny when the abuse had occurred in if you like real time. It also made me acutely aware of the importance of the interactions between different voices that people hear)

When the voice of Jenny the child told him she was ready to confront the abuser we decided to make two days available for the confrontation. Jenny arrived one Friday afternoon and we chatted for a couple of hours not about voices or how she was feeling but just relaxing. Then on the Saturday morning we got down to work. Jenny the child voice told the abuser exactly what she felt, she told him that it was him that should have left the family home, that it was he that was the perpetrator and her that was the victim. She old him that she was innocent and that he was guilty, that she had the right to hate him and no longer felt that she was evil. She repeated much of this over the course of the day, every time the abuser voice tried to regain control of the situation Jenny the child would be backed up by Jenny, the grandmother and myself. By the end of that day although we were exhausted we both knew something had changed and that much had now been resolved. Even now though it was not as we expected it to be, there were no great victory celebrations only the quiet that follows any major battle. It was some weeks later before we sat down together to look at what had happened since the day of the confrontation.

Ask the group what they think happened to each of the voices

There had been some remarkable changes in the voices that Jenny was hearing; the abuser voice was no longer dominant though it was still there. We surmised from this that the reason it had not gone completely was that though Jenny had dealt with the abuse she could not become un-abused, that is she could not change what had happened only her response. The grandmother voice had now become dominant and that was okay for Jenny as it was as always a positive voice. It was the disappearance of the child voice that was the most significant change and we concluded that this had happened due to the end of the need for Jenny to disassociate from her past. Indeed we believe that Jenny the adult and Jenny the child voice became Jenny the person. These changes have now remained constant in her life for over twelve years, without doubt Jenny has reclaimed her life, and she has in fact recovered.

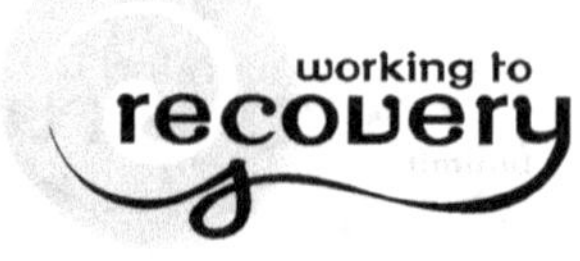

On the role of the worker in this process Coleman states;

"My role in this process was minimal I played only a bit part it was Jenny who did all the hard work I only created the space in which she could do this work. It is clear to me that this is one of the main roles that professionals can play when working with clients. Clients who are working through complex recovery journeys require this type of support to enable them to complete their journeys successfully. I cannot believe that this is an impossible shift for professionals to make indeed I would argue that many already do these types of interventions and that many more wish to. My only advice for professionals is simple, do it".

As we work with people around their voices we gain the confidence that enables us to practice effectively. There is no substitute for working with voice hearers and their voices, it is impossible to learn everything in the classroom situation.

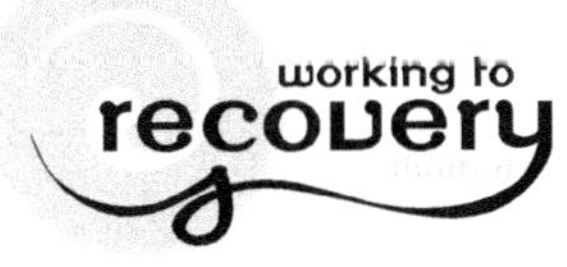

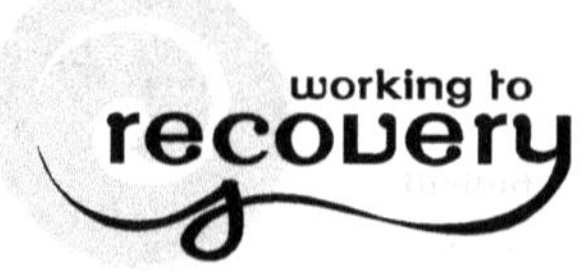

Developing Practice

In this final section we shall explore ways in which we can develop effective ways of working with voice hearers. It is not possible to go into great depth in this manual rather we will touch on various techniques available and point you in the right direction to obtain the information that you need to develop your skills further. The following ways of working will be explored

1.   The Maastricht Interview Schedule

2.   Working with Voices II

3.   Voice Dialoguing

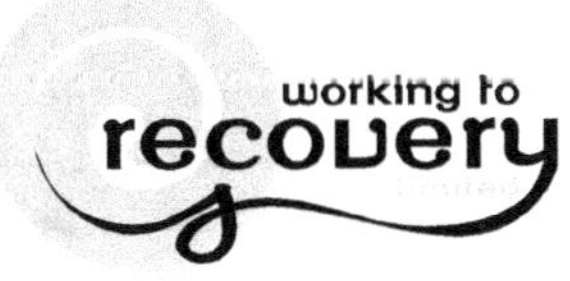

Romme and Escher, primarily as a research tool, developed the Maastricht interview schedule though before long its usefulness as a practice tool was recognised. Many service users have described the interview, on its own as a turning point in their lives. The main reason for this in our opinion is the structure of the interview, which encourages the voice hearer to explore their experience in great depth.

The interview is in twelve sections. The first section focuses on the voice hearer's perception of their experience. The second section explores the characteristics of the person's voices in much the same way as voice profiling. The third section of the interview concentrates on the history of the voice hearer's voices. In the fourth section the voice hearer is encouraged to explore any triggers that are associated with increased voices activity. It is only when you start on the fifth section of the interview that the focus moves to the content of the voices. This makes a great deal of sense in that by this point the interviewer should have created a degree of safety within the process that will allow the voice hearer to tackle the more difficult questions.

The sixth section focuses on the influence that voices have over the voice hearer. In part seven of the interview the voice hearer is asked to explore their interpretation and their thoughts around the origin of the voices. Section eight focuses on the relationship the voice hearers has with their voices especially in terms of power and control. Section nine explores the different types of coping strategies that a voice hearer might use. It is only when you reach section ten that the interviewer starts to ask questions about the voice hearer's childhood. Often this would happen in the second meeting by which time given the nature of the interview a trusting relationship.

The eleventh part of the interview is about any interventions that the voice hearer has had in order to help them deal with their voices. The last part of the interview looks at the voice hearer's social network and their (the social network) understanding of the voices.

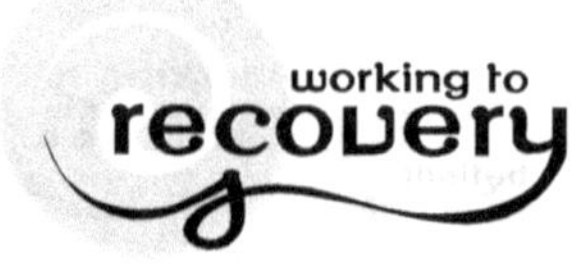

There is no doubt that this tool is a great help to both the worker and the voice hearer. We have included a full copy of the Maastricht Interview Schedule on the CD Rom that accompanies this manual.

Why Talk With Challenging Voices?

Many people who hear challenging voices have found that a turning point in coping with the experience is finding different ways of talking with and understanding them. Exploring the voice's motives and discovering different ways of relating to them can help change the relationship between the voice-hearer and their voices. Techniques derived from various psychological and dramatic traditions (e.g. Gestalt, Voice Dialogue, Transactional Analysis, Psychodrama) have used chairs to act out different roles and relationships in order to help people resolve conflicts and reclaim power in their lives. For the last ten years, a growing number of individuals have adapted this method to use with voice hearing. We came together to write this so that others may try the technique as an aid for coping with negative, distressing voices.

Many people already engage and speak with their voices, and stances can vary from argumentative:
Voice: "You're a failure"
Person: "If I'm a failure what does that make you?"

To challenging:

Voice: "These people don't like you"
Person: "Haven't you got anything better to say?"

To submissive:

Voice: "You shouldn't go out tonight"
Person: "All right then, I won't."

Many voice-hearers experience their voices as a powerful, all-consuming influence - as if they have to obey everything they say, that the voices tell the ultimate truth. Voices can also threaten the voice-hearer with "punishments" for not obeying their commands, either to the person themselves or to friends and family. In our approach, which is derived from a technique known as "Voice Dialogue", we try to explore the motives of the voices so that the person can find new strategies to cope with them. Working with voices in this way can create a more independent position from which an individual can make his/her own choices. Some voices can even become supportive.

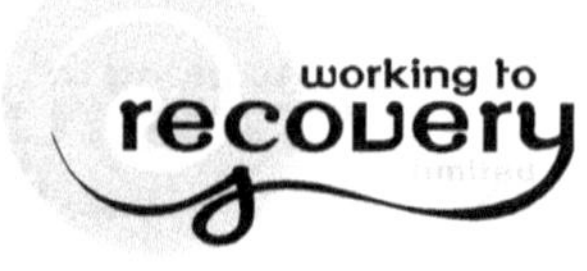

1. This method does not focus on voices as a symptom of "illness": nor does it concentrate on discovering what is "wrong" with the person.

2. It offers a neutral but strong attitude to work with voices - acceptance is the core of the technique.

3. It offers a positive model for the existence of voices.

4. It helps develop increased awareness, objectivity and a more productive relationship between voices and voice-hearer.

5. By definition voice hearing is very lonely experience. Allowing others to "hear" the voices is empowering, liberating and a source of considerable support. In turn, it also affords professionals, friends and family some valuable insight into the reality of a person's voice-hearing experience.

The Theory Behind The Technique: "Voice Dialogue"

This method of working with voices was inspired by a technique known as 'Voice Dialogue' (Stone & Stone, 1993). The name is slightly misleading, as the word 'voice' doesn't actually refer to voices that people hear, but to different aspects of one's personality. According to this model, every person has different 'selves': so-called 'sub-personalities', each with its own way of perceiving the world, its own personal history, emotional reactions and opinions on how we should live our lives. These selves help us cope with difficult situations. For example, the dominant selves want us to succeed in life, and expect us to do whatever a social situation demands. We learn these adaptations very early in life, and our selves stick to what is learned to survive. Our dominant selves push away our more vulnerable parts and these (what is called "disowned" selves) become hidden and unable to play a significant role.

The selves are organised in opposites. For example, if you were brought up with the rule "children should be seen and not heard" you may develop a dominant self that strongly wants to please everybody and focuses on doing whatever is necessary to be liked. The opposite self (the self that wants to ask questions and challenge people, even it means risking rejection) is pushed away by this stronger "Pleaser" self, which craves approval and avoids rejection. A person with selves organised like this doesn't dare to ask questions for fear of rejection. They no longer have a choice between asking for something they need and neglecting what their own needs are.

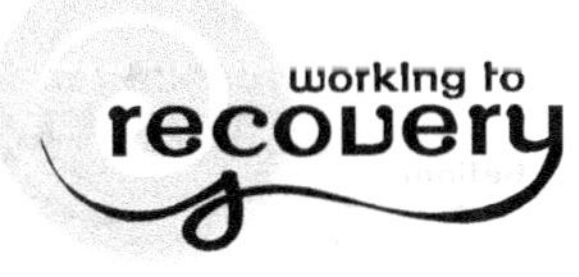

The person has adapted to the rule that was prevalent in history. Originally the organisation of the selves was beneficial to cope with situations in daily life. But in life circumstances change and these selves stay fixated in their originally adaptive roles. So later in life, in other situations, with other people and other needs, the organisation of the selves can prevent you from adaptation. Mostly we are not aware of this process. In the practice of Voice Dialogue, the interviewer (who is not called a 'therapist' but a facilitator') helps you explore these different selves by asking them, one after another, simple questions. The facilitator asks you to concentrate on a self (e.g. the 'pleaser' the 'inner child', the 'leader') and go into the energy of this particular self by standing in a different place in the room. This is a physical demonstration that you are speaking from a different part of yourself.

This specific aspect of the self is then questioned about its function in the person's life, and it is an exciting experience when this self is questioned in such a respectful way. The facilitator elaborates no pressures to change, just expresses their curiosity and desire to acknowledge the presence and individuality of this particular self. The self experiences this acknowledgement and expresses feelings and emotions, like a real person. There will be no discussion or opposing views from the side of the facilitator: the self simply expresses itself without limitations.

Finally, the facilitator asks if the self has any advice for the person, then thanks it and asks the person to return to their original seat and reflect on what happened. Mostly people express surprise, and a sense of increased understanding about how this aspect of them self works in daily life.
(Taken from a training manual on voice dialoguing by Rufus May, Dirk Corstens and Eleanor Longden to be published in 2008)

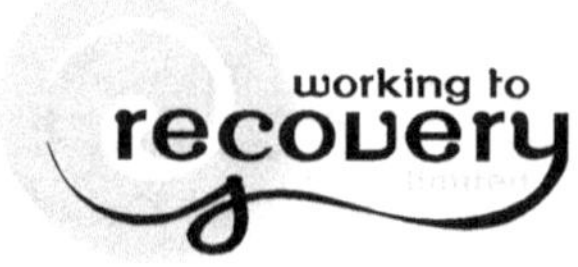

In their workbook Coleman and Smith have developed a tool that allows the voice hearer and worker to engage with the voice hearing experience in a way that allows the voice hearer to take control.

The following is taking from the introduction.

Although we talk about voices throughout we believe that you can mostly apply these principles to visions (seeing voices as we like to sometimes think) and other unusual experiences like feeling or smelling things, if these other experiences are true to you then substitute the words.

Hearing voices does not mean you are sick or ill 4% of the population hear voices, voice hearing is however commoner amongst people who are labeled as mentally ill and so we have little doubt that voices in themselves may not be the problem but they can for some people cause them to have problems that might be described as "Illnesses" Voice hearing in itself is not generally the problem for most people we meet although it may contribute to your problems. Often it is your relationship with your voices, how you interpret them, what they make you believe and how they effect or interfere with your life that may lead to you feeling that you need help, the metaphor illness may be helpful at times in your life but also it can in itself be the problem. Once you are determined to be ill it can be hard to live your life instead of your label and it is certainly hard to prove that you are not ill.

Following a process that helps you reclaim your life!

This book follows a process that many people have described as their natural response to reclaiming their life after being diagnosed as ill and being troubled by unusual experiences. Mike has researched this process and has written widely about it and Ron has lived it. We both believe that recovery is a personal concept and is a journey rather than an event. That said however we believe that as a journey there can be short cuts, there are different routes you can follow and there are people and places along the road that can be positive and negative. We have a rather simple view of recovery, which is "reclaiming your life", so we do not believe that you have to stop hearing voices to recover nor do we believe that there is a right and wrong way, just different paths that lead you to the same place.

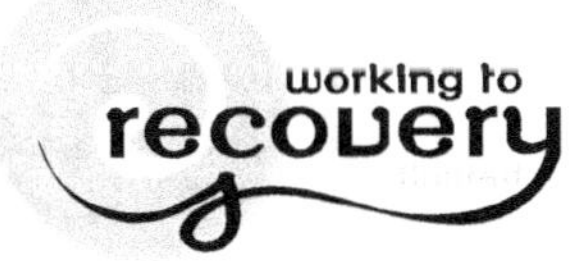

Identifying your experiences

Identifying your experiences in your own words and as you see them   Many people do not fully know, nor are able to share their voice hearing experience, often realising that you are not alone with this experience can be beneficial and recognising for yourself what you are dealing with and putting it into perspective can help.

Exploring your experiences

Looking in depth at your experiences and looking beyond yourself to others and their reactions. We will also look at the relationships you have with your voices, the influence they have over you and how it affects you living your life and what control you do or do not have. This may be the first time you have explored your experiences. This travelling of new ground can be hard both for you and the person who is working with you. I hope it can completely change the way you and others around you view your experiences.

Understanding your Experiences

This is for you, and with your permission a chosen person, to begin to understand and to put into context your experiences.   It aims to clarify your beliefs and to help you make decisions about how you want to move forward together.

Moving on

This phase is about accepting if you want to, and making choices about how you want to cope and live with your voices. It is also about developing strategies for you to take control in your life and for some getting back your life as you want it.   There are a number of coping mechanisms and strategies you can acquire from other people and there is no right way, just the way for you today. This can involve developing an action plan to deal with your experience. Most professionals are required to plan and record what they do for you. You can use this to help you, if you choose, when working with

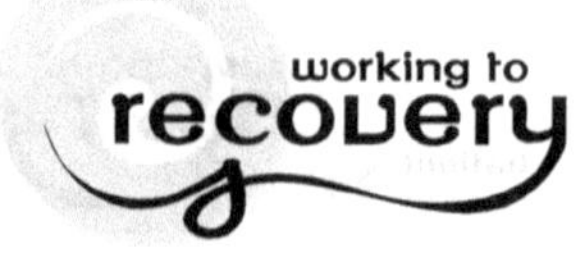

professionals. This plan should be focused around your experiences and how you understand them, and should work to your goals-nobody else's.

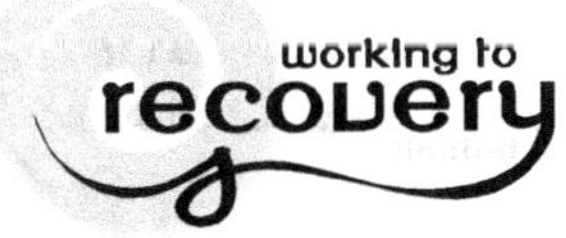

Often when we work through issues around voices we start by identifying the problem, in this edition of the workbook we have turned this on its head and will start by looking at what you want from the process. This is because we have concluded that having dreams and objectives at the beginning of the process gives us a much greater incentive to move forward. Once you know your dreams it is our hope that by working through the workbook you will end up developing an action plan that will allow you to take control of your experience and to live your life.

Creating your Future

There are numerous ways in which you can start planning your goals for the future, we would suggest that you use a technique called mapping. Mapping is a technique that allows you to explore in a focused way where you want to be in your life, how you will get there, what you need to get there, who you need to help you get there and what the pitfalls on your journey might be, we will walk through this at the end of the book.

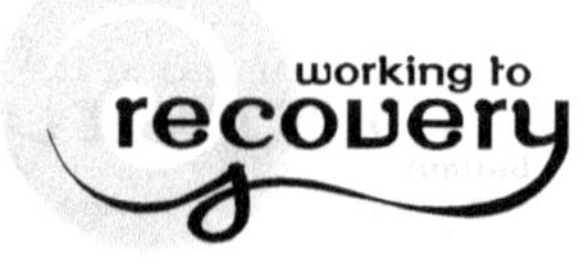

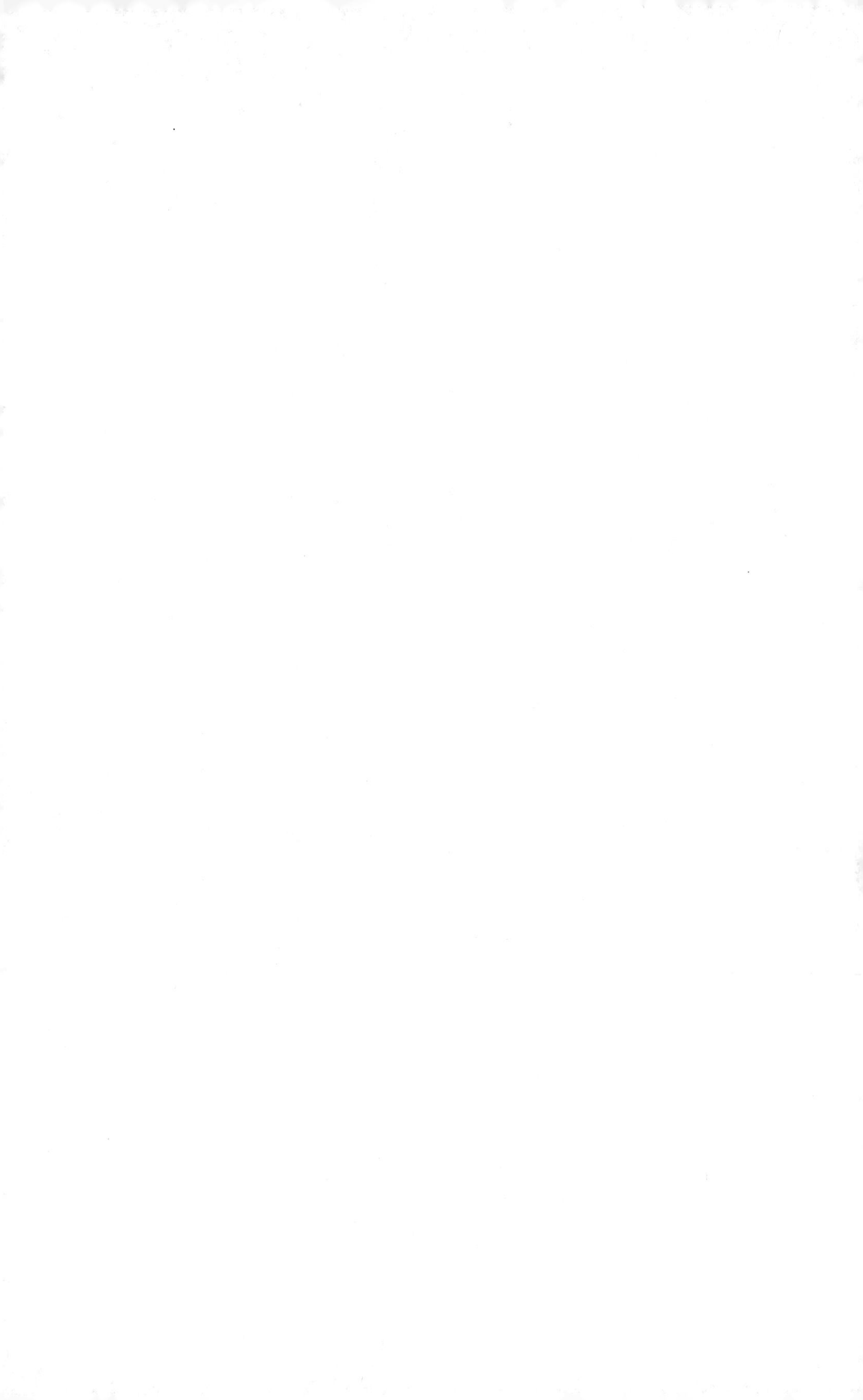